THE GRATITUDE JOURNAL
FOR WOMEN

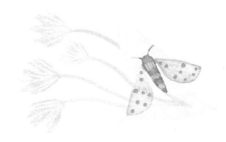

ILLUSTRATIONS BY

Katie
Vernon

TEXT BY

Katherine
Furman

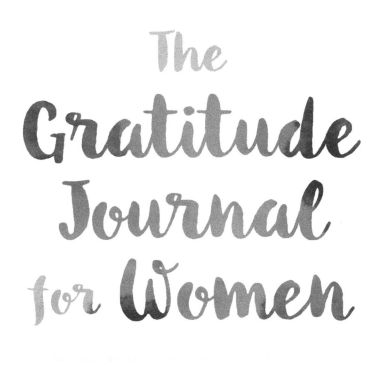

The Gratitude Journal for Women

FIND HAPPINESS AND PEACE
IN **5** MINUTES A DAY

ALTHEA
PRESS

Describe a friend and all the attributes they have that make you glad to know them.

Little things in our daily routine can feel like magic if they bring us joy—a perfect cup of coffee, putting on some cushy slippers, literally stopping to smell the roses. What is your magic moment?

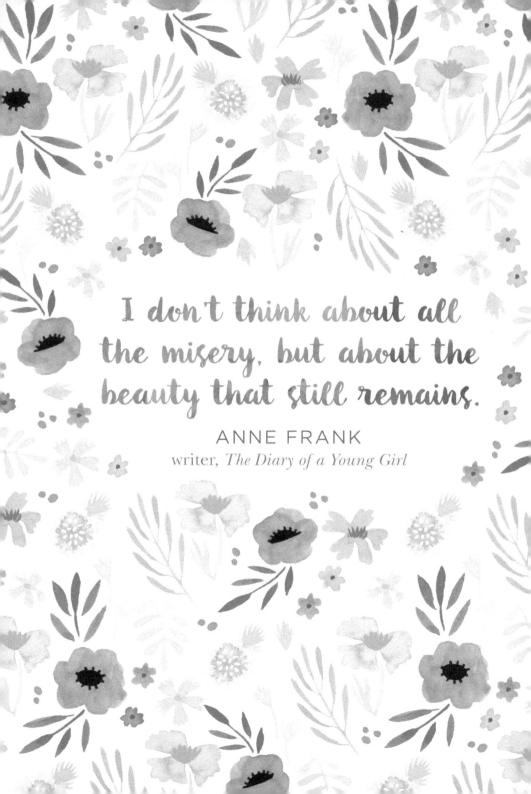

I don't think about all the misery, but about the beauty that still remains.

ANNE FRANK

writer, *The Diary of a Young Girl*

We walk around with long to-do lists in our heads, of things and people we need to take care of. It's easy to forget we take care because we love. List a few of your responsibilities and why you love them.

List at least three things you're really looking forward to, from something as big as a vacation to as small as a scoop of ice cream.

Get a life in which you are generous. Look around at the azaleas making fuchsia star bursts in spring; look at a full moon hanging silver in a black sky on a cold night. And realize that life is glorious, and that you have no business taking it for granted.

ANNA QUINDLEN writer,
A Short Guide to a Happy Life

Feeling gratitude isn't born in us—it's something we are taught, and in turn, we teach our children.

JOYCE BROTHERS writer and psychologist

Change is the one thing you can count on. What is a big transition you've experienced, either by yourself or with a family member, and what good came of it (even if it was hard at the time)?

There are people in the world we don't like, but have to see. Focusing on the negatives can make a bad relationship even harder, while keeping in mind whatever good is there can help ease interactions. Hard as it may be, list the good things about someone you dread seeing.

She has the gift of accepting her life . . .

JHUMPA LAHIRI writer, *The Namesake*

What are you most grateful for today, at this very moment?

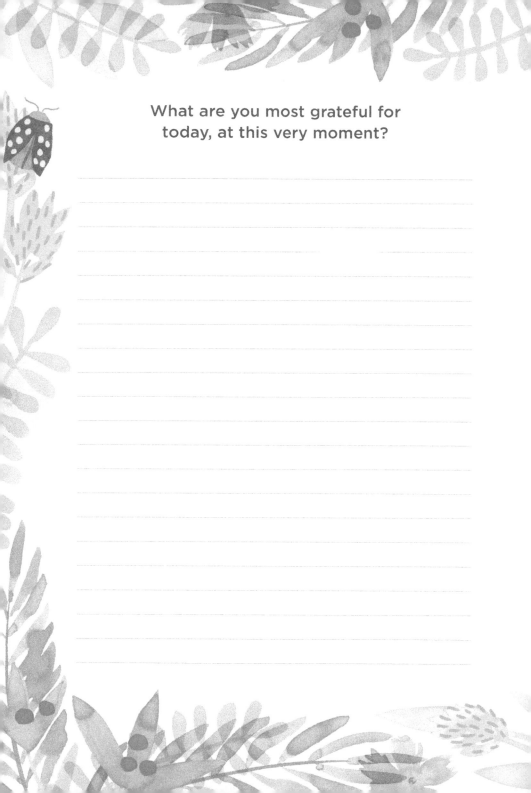

What gift have you given yourself that you are most grateful for?

We are all more blind to what we have
than to what we have not.

AUDRE LORDE writer and activist, *Sister Outsider*

Think about what is most challenging in your life right now and name as many positive aspects of it that you can.

What lesson from childhood are you
really glad you learned early on?

The direct experience of the consciousness of love is gratitude. Gratitude is the process of recognizing what is true. Gratitude is an act of awareness. Without awareness, there is no recognition of anything and, therefore, no love of anything.

TAE YUN KIM writer, speaker, and martial arts instructor, *Seven Steps to Inner Power*

What part of your body are you most grateful for, and why?

Hardships have a way of making us stronger once we emerge from the other side. Write about something that was difficult while it happened, and how you're fiercer now that you've endured it.

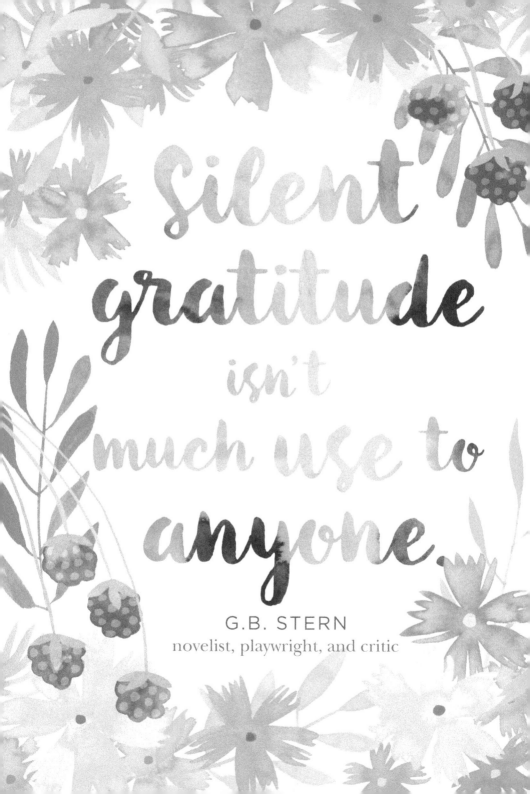

silent gratitude isn't much use to anyone.

G.B. STERN
novelist, playwright, and critic

What do you have that you absolutely can't live without? List every single detail of how and why you adore it.

List three things you are grateful for today.

Unless we learn the lesson of self-appreciation and practice it, we shall spend our lives imitating other people and deprecating ourselves.

AIDA OVERTON WALKER

actor, singer, dancer, and choreographer

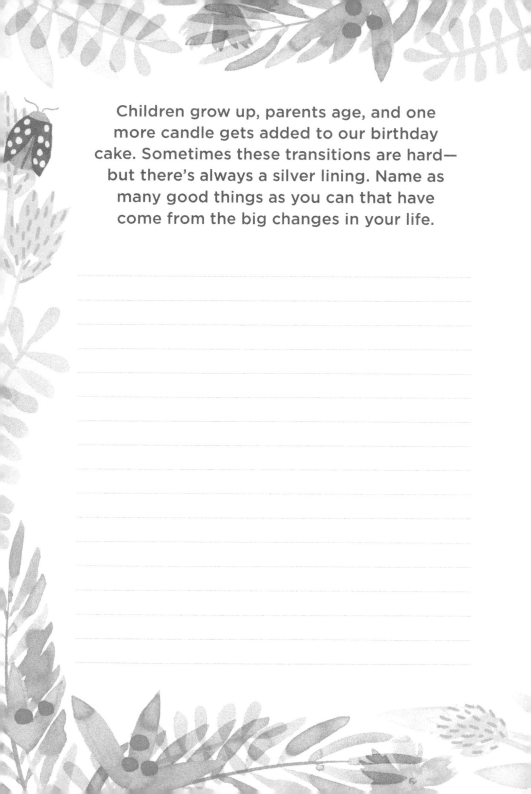

Children grow up, parents age, and one more candle gets added to our birthday cake. Sometimes these transitions are hard—but there's always a silver lining. Name as many good things as you can that have come from the big changes in your life.

What's one thing you're grateful for this year that you didn't have last year?

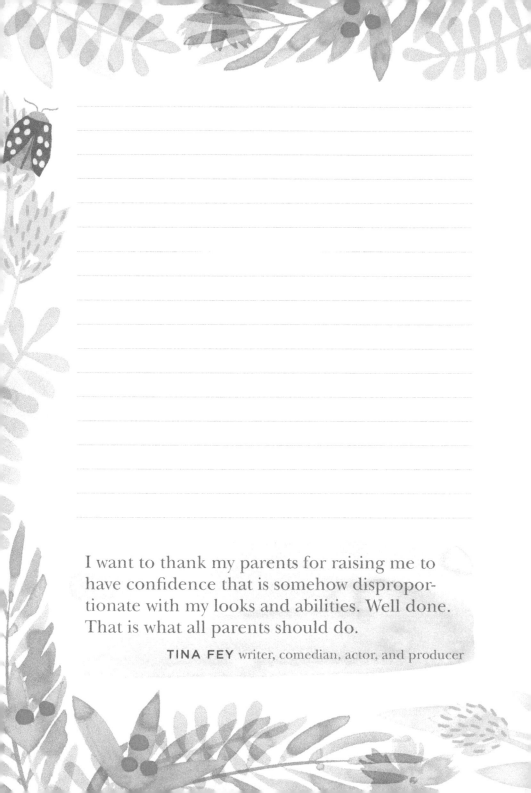

I want to thank my parents for raising me to have confidence that is somehow disproportionate with my looks and abilities. Well done. That is what all parents should do.

TINA FEY writer, comedian, actor, and producer

Mantras are quick statements we can repeat often, in our mind or aloud, to remind us of our values and beliefs— for example, "There are many wondrous things in the world. I am grateful for them, and they fill my heart with joy." Write a few of your own mantras on gratitude.

List what you love about the work you do. Remember that work can be a job, a chore, an art, caretaking, or anything else you put effort into.

Before transition, however unexpected it might be, you could just possibly be granted a moment of centeredness, mindfulness, even a split second of real peace. Peace that comes from gratitude for whatever life you have lived on this astounding Earth.

ALICE WALKER writer and activist, *The Cushion in the Road*

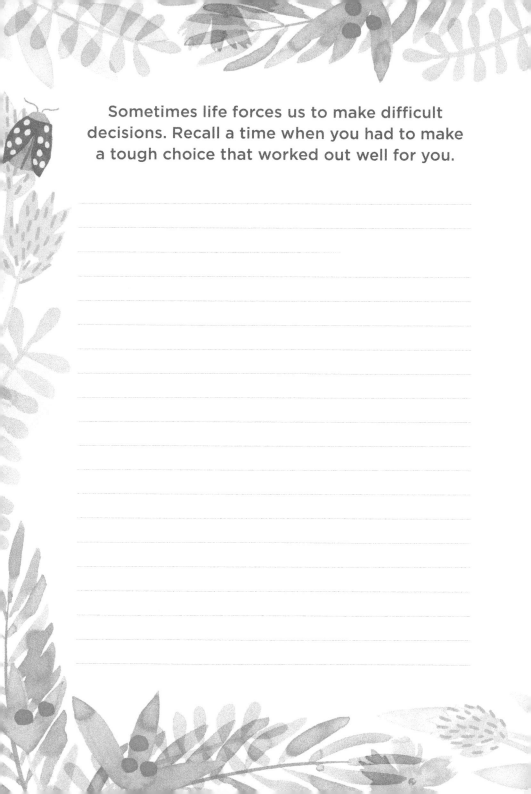

Sometimes life forces us to make difficult decisions. Recall a time when you had to make a tough choice that worked out well for you.

Describe a beautiful day you spent outside. Remember as many details as you can about how it felt, physically and emotionally.

We often take for granted the very things
that most deserve our gratitude.

CYNTHIA OZICK writer

List what you've received from
a parent, tangible or otherwise,
that you are grateful for.

Think about a moment when you felt truly grateful. Describe it in as much detail as you can—from where you were, to who was there, to how you felt.

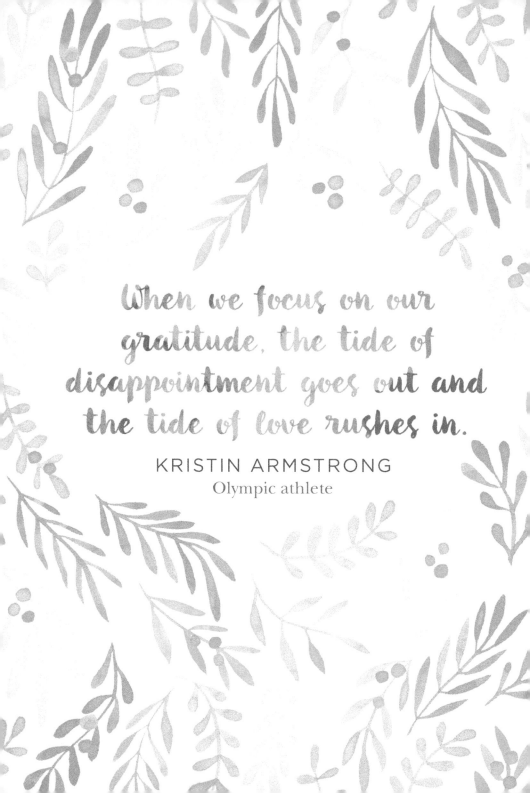

When we focus on our gratitude, the tide of disappointment goes out and the tide of love rushes in.

KRISTIN ARMSTRONG
Olympic athlete

Write about a small kindness from a stranger
that brightened your day (past or present).

List each person in your family and one thing
you are either grateful for or something
about each that makes you happy.

Let us swell with gratitude and allow it to overwhelm us. It isn't as cliché as we make it; life truly is short. Let's spend it all lavishly wallowing in gratitude.

GRACE GEALEY actor

Sunlight through a window, a revitalizing shower, a hot cup of tea. The pleasure of these early-in-the-day events are easily overlooked in our busy lives. What part of your morning routine are you most grateful for?

What is the absolute best thing about the place you live?

It has been said that life has treated me harshly; and sometimes I have complained in my heart because many pleasures of human experience have been withheld from me . . . if much has been denied me, much, very much, has been given me.

HELEN KELLER writer, educator, and social activist, *The Open Door*

The beauty of the natural world, from a single petal to an entire forest, can make us so joyful to be alive. What aspects of nature make you experience that soaring feeling?

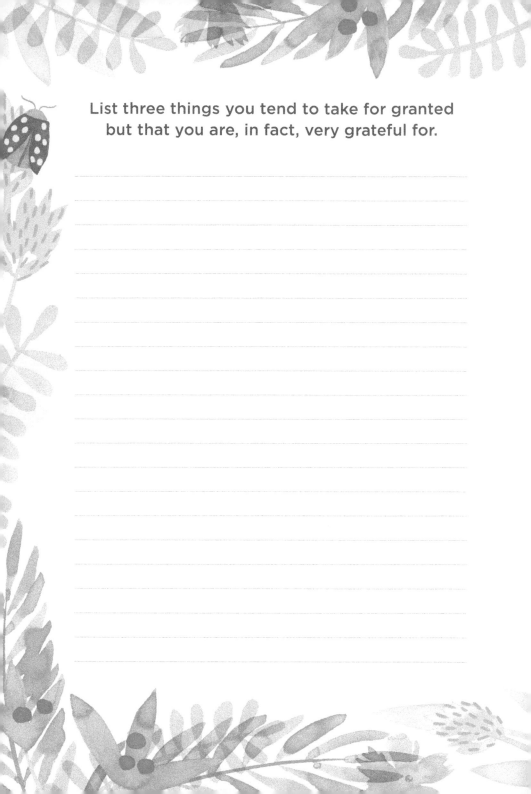

List three things you tend to take for granted
but that you are, in fact, very grateful for.

There is so much that I am grateful for today!
I have arms! I have legs! I have feet! I can
speak! I can think! I can hear! I can see!

IYANLA VANZANT speaker, writer,
and life coach, *Every Day I Pray*

Describe a family member or friend who
is always there for you no matter what.
Include the things they've helped you with.

The modern world is full of marvels! Why are you glad to live in the current age?

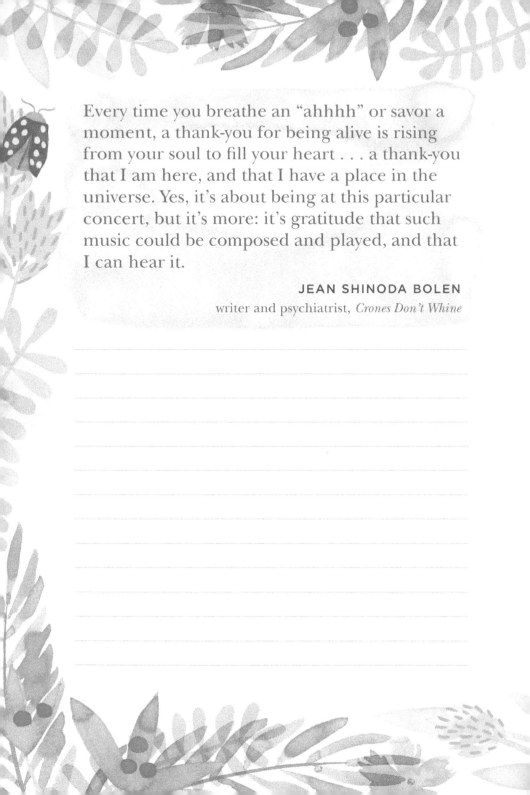

Every time you breathe an "ahhhh" or savor a moment, a thank-you for being alive is rising from your soul to fill your heart . . . a thank-you that I am here, and that I have a place in the universe. Yes, it's about being at this particular concert, but it's more: it's gratitude that such music could be composed and played, and that I can hear it.

JEAN SHINODA BOLEN
writer and psychiatrist, *Crones Don't Whine*

Look around you and list everything
you see that you appreciate.

Look in the mirror and list everything
you see that you are grateful for.

What a
wonderful
life
I've had!
I only wish
I'd realized it
sooner.

SIDONIE-GABRIELLE COLETTE
French novelist

What does gratitude feel like to you?

Despite the pain of losing something you love deeply, it is better to have loved something and lost it than to never have had it in the first place. Think of something you have loved and lost and write about why, even with the hurt, you're glad for the experience.

Ingratitude calls forth reproaches, as gratitude brings fresh kindnesses.

MADAME DE SÉVIGNÉ writer

List three things about your home
that you truly, deeply love.

Think about the people who love you most. Imagine how they see you. List the things about you they are grateful for.

Only a just appreciation of things will enable us to possess them in tranquility, or console ourselves for their loss.

MADAME SWETCHINE Russian mystic

Reflect on one really difficult action
you have to take and one thing about
doing it you can appreciate.

It's easy to put off something difficult that we need to do: organize a messy room, start a job search, confront someone who is hurting us. What is something you have been meaning to do? Why will you be grateful when it's done?

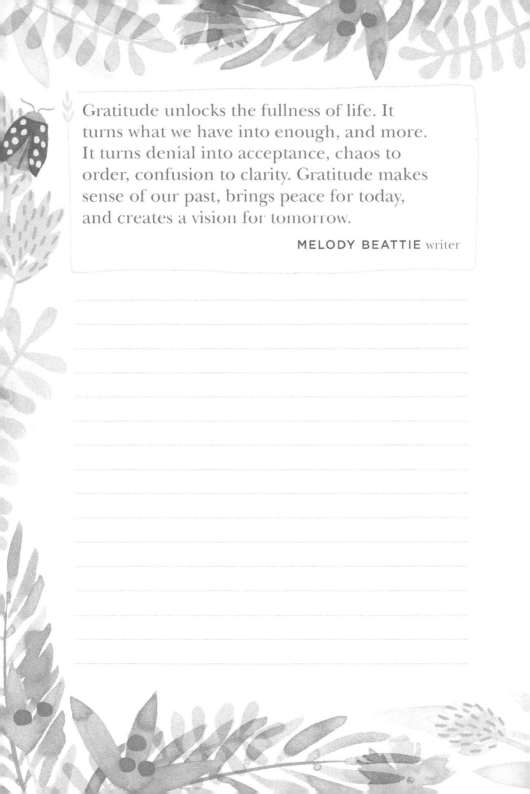

Gratitude unlocks the fullness of life. It turns what we have into enough, and more. It turns denial into acceptance, chaos to order, confusion to clarity. Gratitude makes sense of our past, brings peace for today, and creates a vision for tomorrow.

MELODY BEATTIE writer

Describe a *really* good memory.
Try to relive how it felt, what it looked
like, even what it smelled like. Capture
the details as vividly as you can.

List every trait you have that you are grateful for.

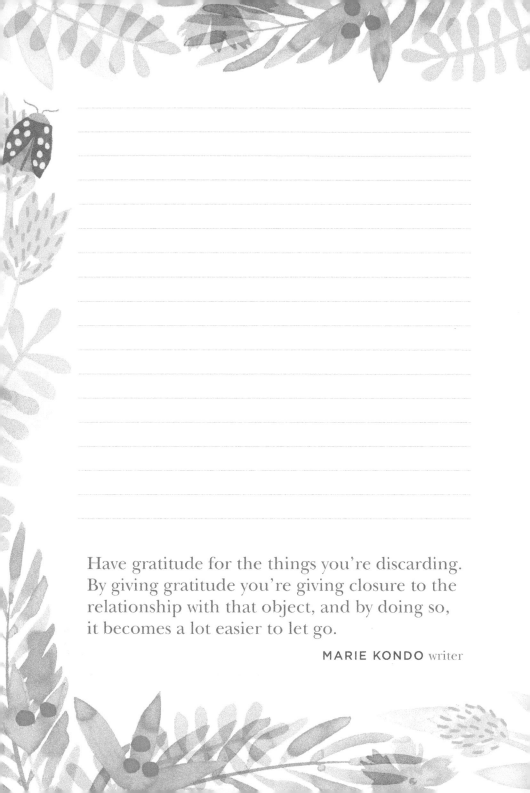

Have gratitude for the things you're discarding. By giving gratitude you're giving closure to the relationship with that object, and by doing so, it becomes a lot easier to let go.

MARIE KONDO writer

Who in your family are you most grateful for, and why?

Write about the time a friend really came through for you and how it made you feel.

_____

_____

_____

_____

_____

_____

_____

_____

_____

_____

_____

_____

_____

_____

_____

_____

_____

_____

_____

_____

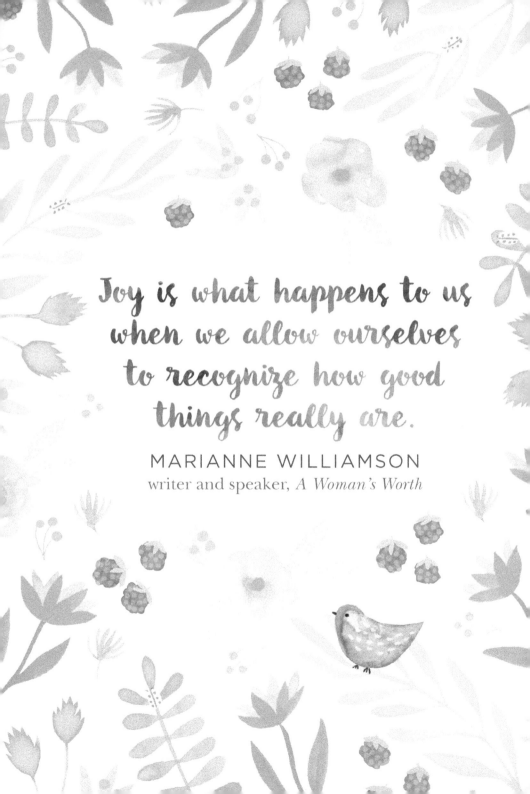

Joy is what happens to us when we allow ourselves to recognize how good things really are.

MARIANNE WILLIAMSON
writer and speaker, *A Woman's Worth*

Think about your day and find three
small things you'd normally overlook
but that you're glad happened.

Art and literature can be inspiring. Think about a favorite piece of art—a painting, a book, a movie, music, anything that means *art* to you—and describe your appreciation for it.

We learned about gratitude and humility—
that so many people had a hand in our success,
from the teachers who inspired us to the
janitors who kept our school clean . . . and we
were taught to value everyone's contribution
and treat everyone with respect.

MICHELLE OBAMA writer, lawyer, and former First Lady

We've all had happy accidents in our lives—a chance meeting, arriving for an appointment at the wrong time only to have it work out in our favor, or maybe something as simple as getting the wrong order at a coffee shop and discovering a new favorite. What is your happiest accident?

Which food or meal are you most grateful for? Describe it in delicious detail.

. . . we really live in a small world, and we all are affected by everything that happens everywhere. And to look at it less selfishly, we also need to be grateful for the luck of where we're born and how we ended up where we ended up.

NATALIE PORTMAN actor

There are so many inspirational people in the world, both famous and in our day-to-day lives—from doctors to performers to those who keep smiling through everything life throws their way. Describe how someone has inspired you, and why you're glad for that inspiration.

Life is never perfect, but who needs perfect anyway? List some of your flaws and why you appreciate them.

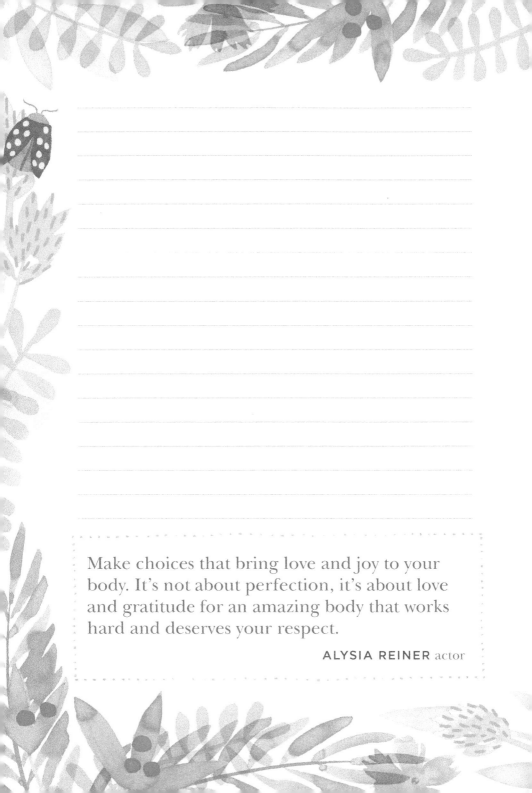

Make choices that bring love and joy to your body. It's not about perfection, it's about love and gratitude for an amazing body that works hard and deserves your respect.

ALYSIA REINER actor

What season do you enjoy the most? List all the things about it you look forward to. Are there new ways you can celebrate that season or get more out of it this year?

What invention has had the biggest
positive effect on your life? Why
are you grateful for it?

I am grateful for the blessings of wealth, but it hasn't changed who I am. My feet are still on the ground. I'm just wearing better shoes.

OPRAH WINFREY talk show host, actor, and producer

Holidays, celebrations, and other traditions can serve as touchstones, marking special times of the year or times in our lives. What tradition are you most grateful for, and why?

Animals have a way of capturing our hearts with their innocence, devotion, and antics. Describe an animal—in your life or from a book or movie—that made you feel grateful for its presence.

Love and gratitude can part seas, move mountains, and create miracles.

RHONDA BYRNE writer and producer, *The Secret*

What skill do you have that you're grateful for? Does it come naturally to you, or did you have to work hard to acquire it?

Wabi-sabi is a Japanese term that refers to finding beauty in imperfection—a gnarled tree made all the more intriguing for its oddness, a space between a friend's two front teeth that makes her face hypnotically gorgeous, a threadbare patch in a favorite pair of jeans. List some wabi-sabi that you're grateful for.

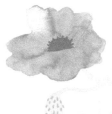

Reflections

Now that you've completed your gratitude journal, you can more easily recognize and appreciate the many things you have to be grateful for. Hopefully, this exploration has also brought you a greater sense of positivity and contentment, which in turn has helped minimize stressors, both big and small.

To bring your gratitude journey full circle and reinforce all the good you've identified on these pages, go back and read your entries. Try to absorb all the gratitude you've expressed as fully as you can. Bring it into your body, your mind, and your heart, and be nourished by it. Being mindful of the people, places, and events in your world that make your heart sing reinforces happiness and calm on a daily basis. You may even find ways to appreciate hardships and trials. Silver linings that you may not have noticed or fully understood before now shine in easy view, bright and gleaming.

Once you have read your entries, ask yourself:

What are the three most important things I learned about myself?

What are the three aspects I wrote about in this journal that I am most grateful for?

Has my outlook on the world changed since I started
keeping this journal? If so, in what ways?
Have I begun to share my gratitude with others?

By revisiting your journal, you may see themes or
patterns you didn't notice while first writing your entries.
You may surprise yourself by what you said. Maybe you
will learn something new about your perspective or how
that perspective has changed through the course of your
writing. The complete picture of your life lived with gratitude will come into focus, which will support and nourish
you as you lean into the future.

Gratitude Going Forward

Just because this journal has come to an end does not mean your newfound—or newly identified—appreciation has to ebb. Pick a few of your favorite prompts and write about them whenever you like. Repeat the mantras you wrote for yourself any time, any place. Read over the pages and draw strength from the many, many things you have to be grateful for, and fortify yourself with the wise words of so many thoughtful women.

Maintaining gratitude is as easy as looking around you, picking one thing you like, and saying, "Thank goodness for that!"

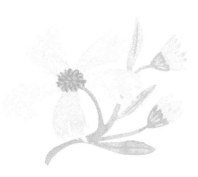

Resources

FOR FURTHER READING ON GRATITUDE, SEE

DeMoss, Nancy Leigh. *Choosing Gratitude: Your Journey to Joy*. Chicago: Moody Publishers, 2009.

Emmons, Robert A. *Thanks! How Practicing Gratitude Can Make You Happier*. New York: Houghton Mifflin Harcourt, 2008.

Fox, Glenn. "What Can the Brain Reveal about Gratitude?" *Greater Good Magazine*, August 4, 2017. greatergood.berkeley.edu/article/item/what_can _the_brain_reveal_about_gratitude.

Harvard Medical School. "Giving Thanks Can Make You Happier." *Harvard Health Publications*. www.health .harvard.edu/healthbeat/giving-thanks-can-make-you -happier.

Hay, Louise L. *Gratitude: A Way of Life*. Carlsbad, CA: Hay House, 1996.

Kaplan, Janice. *The Gratitude Diaries: How a Year Looking on the Bright Side Can Transform Your Life*. New York: Dutton, 2016.

Positive Psychology Program. "What is Gratitude and What is Its Role in Positive Psychology?" February 28, 2017. www.positivepsychologyprogram.com/gratitude-appreciation.

Ryan, M. J. *Attitudes of Gratitude: How to Give and Receive Joy Every Day of Your Life.* Berkeley, CA: Conari Press, 1999.

Sacks, Oliver. *Gratitude.* New York: Knopf, 2015.

Wiking, Meik. *The Little Book of Hygge: Danish Secrets to Happy Living.* New York: William Morrow, 2017.

WEBSITES

A Network for Grateful Living: www.gratefulness.org/resource/how-to-practice-gratitude/

Happify Daily: www.my.happify.com/hd/cultivate-an-attitude-of-gratitude/

Oprah Winfrey: www.oprah.com/app/happiness-and-gratitude.html

Positive Psychology Program: www.positivepsychologyprogram.com/gratitude-exercises/

Unstuck: www.unstuck.com/gratitude/

References

Conger, Cristen. "Is There a Link between Gratitude and Happiness?" June 16, 2009. HowStuffWorks.com. science.howstuffworks.com/life/inside-the-mind/ emotions/gratitude-and-happiness1.htm. August 26, 2017.

Emmons, Robert A., and Michael E. McCullough. "Counting Blessings versus Burdens: An Experimental Investigation of Gratitude and Subjective Well-Being in Daily Life." *Journal of Personality and Social Psychology* 84, no. 2 (2003): 377–389. doi:10.1037/0022-3514.84.2.377.

Harvard Medical School. "Giving Thanks Can Make You Happier." *Harvard Health Publications.* www.health .harvard.edu/healthbeat/giving-thanks-can-make-you -happier.

Seligman, Martin E. P., Tracy A. Steen, N. Park, and C. Peterson. "Positive Psychology Progress: Empirical Validation of Interventions." *The American Psychologist* 60, no. 5 (July–August 2005): 410–21. doi:10.1037/0003-066X.60.5.410.

Watkins, Philip C., Kathrane Woodward, Tamara Stone, and Russell L. Kolts. "Gratitude and Happiness:

Development of a Measure of Gratitude, and Relation-
ships with Subjective Well-Being." *Social Behavior
and Personality* 31, no 5. (August 2003): 431–452.
doi.org/10.2224/sbp.2003.31.5.431.

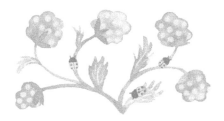

Acknowledgments

For a *Gratitude Journal for Women*, it only makes sense that I thank two of the amazing, strong, and inspiring women in my life—my mom and my daughter. Thank you, mom, for believing in and encouraging me throughout my life. Thank you, Juniper, for pushing me to grow in ways I never imagined.

— Katie Vernon

There are so many people who have helped make this journal come to life, and I am grateful to each and every one. To my business partner, Ashley Prine, for being utterly indefatigable. To my husband, for being a singular man who can find fun anywhere and in anything. To my parents for believing I could do absolutely anything— warranted or not. To Marilyn Kretzer for introducing me to Callisto Media. And to Susan Randol and Elizabeth Castoria for being not only consummate professionals but also super fun to work with.

—Katherine Furman

About the Illustrator

KATIE VERNON is an illustrator who has spent most of her life in the Midwest, but whose heart belongs in the mountains. She loves working with inky paints and then arranging and adding detail digitally. She is most thankful for her husband, daughter, and part-dingo dog.

About the Author

KATHERINE FURMAN is a long-time editor and writer of nonfiction. She has worked on countless subjects, from humor to health to history, and she is profoundly grateful for each and every opportunity she's had. She is the cofounder and the editorial director of Tandem Books, a publishing studio, and lives with her husband in Atlantic Highlands, New Jersey.

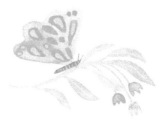

CPSIA information can be obtained
at www.ICGtesting.com
Printed in the USA
BVIIW022226141218
535462BV00019B/73/P